The pH miracle
for Diabetes & Obesity

by Dr. Robert O. Young, Ph.D., D.Sc.

The pH Miracle for Diabetes & Obesity
By Dr. Robert O. Young, Ph.D., D.Sc.

Printed in the United States
1st Printing August 2004
2nd Printing May 2009

For questions or comments,
please email info@DiabetesResearchSociety or call 800.871.1631
Visit http://DiabetesResearchSociety.org/

No information contained herein is meant to replace the advice of a qualified health-care practitioner. For proper diagnosis, consult your doctor. The data and opinions appearing in this book are for informational purposes only. Robert O. Young Ph.D, D.Sc. and Shelley Redford Young do not offer medical advice, and he encourages readers to seek advice from qualified health professionals.

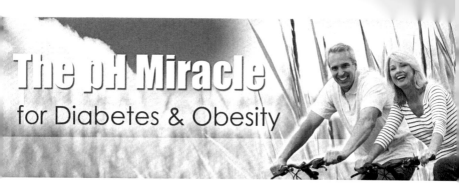

The pH Miracle
for Diabetes & Obesity

ABOUT THE AUTHOR

D r. Robert O. Young is recognized as one of the leading research scientists in the world. He holds a degree in microbiology and nutrition. His research has explored the causes of disease and how to help people regain their health and well-being. Dr. Young is also the developer of the new paradigm of human disease, and the discoverer of the etiology of diabetes, cancer and atherosclerosis, amoung other diseases.

As the head of the Robert O. Young Research Center and Health Education foundation, he has gained national recognition for his research into diabetes, cancer, leukemia and AIDS. His proprietary Mycotoxic/Oxidative Stress Test reliably predicts the onset of degenerative conditions. He is also a pioneer in colloidal technology.

Dr. Young is a member of the American Society of Micro-biologists and the American Naturopathic Association. He is a popular speaker at medical and health gatherings all over the world.

TABLE OF CONTENTS

CHAPTER I
INTRODUCTION

Our ancestors would be over-whelmed by the bountiful life we enjoy today. We have literally hundreds of modern conveniences that didn't even exist in their wildest imaginings. While they often struggled to place meager servings of bread on their tables, we have food available on almost every corner. But, according to Marion Nestle, Ph.D., a nutritionist at New York University, that's not necessarily a blessing. Since 1970, food serving sizes have doubled and in some cases quadrupled. In 2000, the U.S. food industry provided about 3,900 calories per person per day, of which the USDA estimated that the average American consumed around 2,750 calories. That's more

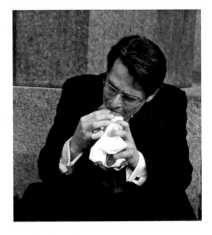

than 500 calories above the recommended 2,200 calories. Yet, even that recommended amount is above the average caloric intake from 20 years ago. That average, according to the USDA, was a meager 1,854 calories.

CHAPTER 2
TOO MANY CALORIES
CAUSE PROBLEMS

The problem doesn't necessarily lie in the accessibility of this great caloric abundance, but rather in the final destination of those excess calories.

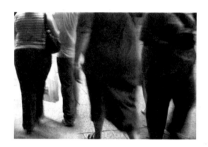

OBESITY

A 1991 report showed that less than 15 percent of the U.S. population was obese. Ten years later, the Centers for Disease Control and Prevention reported a 61 percent increase in obesity. One in three American adults is considered seriously overweight. This is terrible news when you consider that excess weight causes at least 300,000 deaths annually; costs more than $117 billion in healthcare; and increases the risk of developing serious health challenges like diabetes with all of its attending side effects, such as cardiovascular disease, stroke, and cancer-just to name a few.

Unfortunately, it's not just adults who are suffering from this epidemic. In 2001, the Surgeon General reported that 13 percent of young children and 14 percent of adolescents—that's triple the amount from just 20 years ago—are overweight. Early obesity increases the likelihood of adult obesity, and it increases the same health risks that adults face. In fact, in 1999 physicians began to report an alarming increase in the number of children with type II diabetes—a kind of diabetes formerly known as "adult onset diabetes."

DIABETES

This obesity epidemic, however, is just the forerunner of a much more deadly epidemic. "Right behind this obesity epidemic," states James

Hill, Director of the Center for Human Nutrition at the University of Colorado Health Sciences Center, "is a diabetes epidemic, and that is very expensive." Current statistics rank diabetes as the sixth-highest cause of death among Americans. In 1999, there were 68,399 people who died from diabetes. That same year, an additional 141,265 deaths were listed with diabetes as a contributing factor. Those numbers are going to rise incrementally over the next few years as this epidemic runs its course.

Currently, 17 million people have diabetes. Of that group, 151,000 are under the age of 20. The occurrence of type II diabetes is becoming increasingly common, especially among children and adolescents, reports the American Diabetes Association.

What do all these numbers mean? When you consider that diabetics face two times the risk of death compared to non-diabetics, you can see the staggering death toll that this disease will have. But it's not just the diabetic deaths that we need to worry about; diabetics are also at increased risk of heart disease, stroke, blindness, kidney disease, nervous system disease, dental disease, pregnancy complications, and amputation.

Though these epidemics of obesity and diabetes are sweeping the nation, you are not defenseless against them. There are many things that you can—and should—do to help counter the effects of obesity and diabetes. This booklet is geared towards educating you on your options.

CHAPTER 3
BUILDING A HEALTH PLAN

One of the most important things you can do for your health is to practice proper nutrition. No big surprise, right? What may be a surprise is that, though we have an incredible amount of food available, we are not getting the nutrients we need.

In June, 2002, the *Journal of the American Medical Association* (JAMA) reported that the average American diet is sufficient to prevent vitamin deficiency diseases like scurvy. The article continued to state that "recent evidence has shown that suboptimal levels of vitamins, even well above those causing deficiency syndromes, are risk factors for chronic disease such as diabetes, cardiovascular disease, cancer, and osteoporosis. A large proportion of the general population is apparently at increased risk for this reason.... The high prevalence of suboptimal vitamin levels implies that the usual U.S. diet provides an insufficient amount of these vitamins."

The JAMA article went on to provide three suggestions to overcome the dangerous lack of nutrients in our modern diets. The first was to add nutrients into generally consumed foods. The second, which also became their recommendation, was to supplement your diet with a daily multivitamin. The final suggestion was to change the American diet.

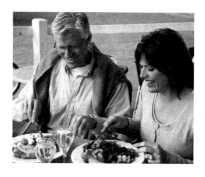

DEVELOP A GOOD DIET PLAN

More and more experts are beginning to see the importance of developing a good diet plan. The USDA's food guide pyramid—the same plan that we all learned about in our school days—is fatally flawed. Fortunately, we're beginning to see the emergence of good food plans. Each of these plans share a common characteristic: they all recommend increased portions of fruits and vegetables.

Recently the American Institute for Cancer Research (AICR) released a new food guide calling for vegetables, fruits, whole grains, and beans to cover two-thirds or more of your plate while animal source foods should cover only one-third. The Healthy Eating Pyramid (developed by Dr. Walter Willet and his colleagues at the Harvard School of Public Health after reviewing the data from the Nurses' Health Study, Physicians' Health Study, and the Health Professionals' Follow-up Study) has similar recommendations, focusing on increased whole-grain foods, plant oils, and vegetables. The AICR's research into their diet recommendations showed that 78 percent of studies on fruits

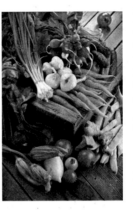

and vegetables and cancer showed a positive, protective effect. Willet's research showed that women adhering to the Healthy Eating Pyramid are 28 percent less likely to suffer from heart disease—that's double the number of adherents to the USDA guidelines.

As a society, we are beginning to see the incredible importance of eating right. Though we still have a long way to go, we are taking a vital step toward improving our health. The growing focus on eating fruits and vegetables will help our nation's health incredibly.

But proper nutrition is only part of the battle. Not only do we need to make sure that our calories aren't empty and void of nutrients, we also need to cut back on the amount of calories that we consume.

Our cornucopia of calories has created the obesity epidemic that now weighs us down. Obesity has long been known to be a major risk factor in developing type II diabetes. Simply put, the more over-weight you are the more danger you are in. Your first step in preventing, treating, and even curing diabetes is to lose any excess weight you may be carrying around.

Easier said than done though, right? Not necessarily. Losing weight can be a matter of changing just a few health practices. We've already discussed one aspect: proper nutri-tion. When you provide your body with what it needs, your body will require less and less food intake. You'll also feel healthier, which will translate into better mental health. All of this means less crav-ings and more activity—the key to any weight-loss plan.

And more activity is a major part of weight loss. You eat food to provide your body with building materials and fuel for activity. It stands to reason, then, that if you increase your activity you will need more fuel. Providing your body with the correct amount of calories will let your body maintain its current size. If you add more acidic calories than what you need, your body will begin to store these excess acids in the extremities of the body, such as the hips, thighs, buttocks, waistline, breast, and brain. The other side is also true and more desirable. If you eat less acidic foods and eat more electron-rich foods and stay active, then you will store less acid on your hips, thighs, buttocks, waistline, breast, and brain, creating a weight loss.

BEGIN AN EXERCISE ROUTINE

That's where exercise comes in. Exercise is activity, and activity means burning fuel and eliminating acidic wastes. Even simple activities like walking can help to move acids out through the pores of the skin by sweating. That's not all; exercise has a whole set of benefits that accompany it. Keeping your body in motion increases brain and heart health. It improves the range of motion for your joints as well as helping in the battle against arthritis. Exercise also increases your lean body mass-your muscles. Muscles are the engines that burn the fuel you eat. The more muscle you have, the higher your fuel requirements will be—meaning you burn more calories both when active and at rest. Finally, exercise helps control stress levels, giving you a forum in which you can release the day's pent-up anxiety.

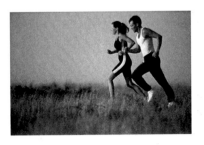

The most pertinent aspect of exercise to the topic at hand, however, is what it can do for the diabetic. In some people, exercise may improve insulin sensitivity and assist in lowering elevated glucose levels, reports the American Diabetic Association. Exercise does this because it increases the demand for oxygen in your body. This increase causes muscles to use more glucose to meet their energy demands. As a result, blood glucose levels drop as more fuel is burned. At the same time, exercise improves the action of insulin in periphery muscles, making it more efficient. This means that your body gets more out of the insulin it produces.

Exercise Can Prevent Diabetes and Obesity

According to a study conducted by the National Institute of Diabetes and Digestive and Kidney Diseases, as many as 10 million Americans who are high risk of type II diabetes can lower their risks of developing the disease through diet and exercise. The study involved 3,234 people who already showed signs of developing type II diabetes. Of those people, those who lost 5 percent - 7 percent of their body weight and walked or performed other moderate physical activity for 30 minutes a day reduced their risk of type II diabetes by 58 percent. The results of the study—which was sponsored by the National Institutes of Health, the American Disabilities Association and others—were so astounding that the study was concluded a year earlier than planned.

Given the amount of information that's our there, it may be hard to understand exactly what you're supposed to do to reap the benefits of exercise. In September 2002, the Institute of Medicine (IOM) issued a report recommending that adults spend at least 60 minutes in moderately intense physical activity every day of the week. This recommendation doubled the daily minimum goal of 30 minutes of physical activity most days of the

week set by the U.S. Surgeon General in 1996—before obesity reached epidemic proportions. The Surgeon General made his recommendation based on a great deal of research that showed that 30 minutes of physical activity most days of the week could reduce your risk of chronic diseases, including heart disease, diabetes, and colon cancer.

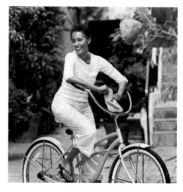

The IOM's recommendation stems from new convincing evidence. The most recent studies show that 30 minutes of activity may not be enough to allow most people to maintain an ideal weight and achieve maximum health benefits. Because most people in the United States are consuming more calories and getting heavier, more exercise is needed in order to offset this excess caloric intake.

So, there you have it. If you're getting the right amount of calories, 30 minutes a day of moderate activity is sufficient. However, if you're eating more than your body requires, you'll need to spend more time on the treadmill each day.

Simply put, practice good health habits and be active for at least 30 minutes every day and you'll stand a strong chance of preventing, treating, and even curing diabetes.

Tips for Safe Exercising

Adding exercise to your lifestyle is very important. Here are some tips to make sure you exercise safely if you are diabetic:

• Check your blood glucose level before and after exercising. You need to know if your level is too high to

exercise safely, or if you need to take action before exercising to prevent hypoglycemia. Consult your doctor about whether you should eat a snack or change your medication dose before exercising.

• Wait one to two hours to exercise after eating a meal to best avoid hypoglycemia.

• Avoid jarring or straining activities, especially if you have retinopathy. Also avoid activities that involve bearing down (such as handball or heavy weight lifting). These activities can cause damage to the fragile blood vessels of the eye.

• Choose the right footwear. Have a thorough foot examination before starting an exercise program.

• Avoid repetitive weight-bearing activities, like basketball, if you have severe loss of sensation. Biking or swimming would be better.

• Drink plenty of fluids. Dehydration can hinder your body's ability to handle glucose.

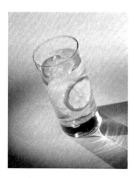

• Have a thorough heart exam before beginning exercise if your family history reveals a propensity toward high cholesterol and/or triglycerides, or an elevated danger of heart attacks, or if you have autonomic neuropathy,

(Adapted from "How much do you know about exercising safely?" Woodrum, J. Diabetes Self-Management, March/April 2002; 19(2) :80, 83)

CHAPTER 4
THE TRUTH ABOUT EXERCISE

Before we move on, there's another aspect of exercise that we should look at. There is an idea touted in the fitness and body-building world that in order to build strength, size, and/or endurance you need to go to the threshold of pain. We've all heard the saying, "No pain, No gain." This philosophy can be hazardous to your health.

A RECIPE FOR DISASTER

Anatomically and physiologically the body is an incredible machine that is designed to move. In order to make a single movement, the body needs energy. That energy is found in our foods and used by the anatomical elements that make up every living cell.

When your car brns or ferments fuel to create energy, a toxin or acid is released called carbon monoxide.

When your body's anatomical elements burn or ferment foods to release energy, the same thing happens. The toxin created is called carbon dioxide.

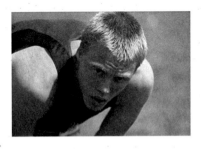

For example, when a sprinter is running a 100-meter race, he or she is burning sugar for energy producing the less toxic acid carbon dioxide which is expelled through the lungs. When the sprinter takes in less oxygen than is needed, he or she becomes oxygen deficient. The mode of energy production changes from respiration (meaning in the presence of oxygen) to fermentation (meaning in the absence of oxygen). Fermentation creates a more toxic acid:

lactic acid. Unlike carbon dioxide, which is expelled out of the body, lactic acid is expelled into the surrounding tissues. This is what causes pain. Anytime you experience or feel aches, pain, or suffer from irritation or inflammation, you are feeling the effect of acid. Therefore, acid equals pain, and pain equals acid.

When you exercise to exhaustion you are creating excess acids that lead to all sickness and disease—including obesity and diabetes. Acids burn and break down cells, which in turn causes a rise in blood sugar. This rise in blood sugar can be devastating to diabetics and is the reason why exercising to exhaustion—or anaerobic exercise—can be hazardous to your health. The ideology "No pain, No gain" is a scientific illusion. It should actually say, "With pain (acid), no healthy gain."

It is important to realize that the principal reason for exercising is to eliminate acids from the body via the lungs through respiration or the skin through perspiration. That is why we have two lungs instead of one, and 3,500 perspiratory pores in our skin per square inch.

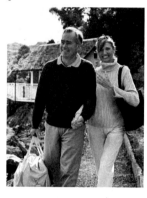

Exercise moves acids through these two elimination organs, reducing endogenous acidity in order to maintain the integrity of all your cells. When your internal environment is alkaline, your cells are stronger and healthier. When your cells are stronger and healthier, your muscles are stronger and healthier, your heart is stronger and healthier, and your pancreas is stronger and healthier. In fact, every organ throughout your body benefits and can function at its optimal level in a balanced pH environment without pain.

A *Newsweek* article published May 19, 2003 stated that pain is the number one reason Americans visit the doctor at an economic cost of $100 billion a year. Over 10 million children in America suffer from chronic and acute pain that ultimately contributes to the increase in childhood diabetes. Why? The cause is over-acidity in the blood and tissues. This over-acidity is the result of our inverted way of living. It is the cause of cancer. It is the cause of sickness and disease. It is the cause of heart disease. It is the cause of diabetes.

CHAPTER 5
FIVE FOUNDATION STONES OF HEALTHY DIETS

It seems simple enough. Getting the right foods and moderate exercise for at least 30 minutes a day will dramatically affect your risks of developing diabetes. But we're not talking about just affecting your risks. The ultimate goal is to eliminate them. To do that, you need to build a health plan—one that includes daily exercise and proper nutrition. Building that plan also involves applying five foundation stones to your diet.

THE 1ST FOUNDATION STONE: GREEN POWDER DRINK

More and more experts are turning their attention to vegetables, and with just cause. The majority of your body's needs can be met through vegetables. Vitamins, minerals, and even macronutrients like protein, carbohydrates, and fats can all be found in plant foods. But there's more to our green friends than just these nutrients. Plant foods also contain biologically active substances that have proven health benefits, such as:

Chlorophyll

Chlorophyll helps blood to deliver oxygen throughout the body; reduces the binding of acids to DNA; helps break down calcium stones; and, most importantly, provides the foundational anatomical elements—microzyma—for building red blood cells.

Plant Enzymes

Your body uses enzymes for the chemical activities necessary for maintaining life. Plant enzymes, among other activities, aid in digestion. This activity frees your body's enzymes for other activities, giving you more energy and aiding in regeneration.

Phytonutrients

Phytonutrients help prevent diabetes by neutralizing acids and other acidic symptoms such as cardiovascular disease, obesity, hypercholesterolemia, arthritis, osteoporosis, and pancreatic cancer.

Just as an example, here are two great vegetables to include in your diet:

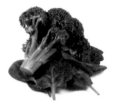

Broccoli

Broccoli is a great source of vitamin C, meeting 97 percent of the recommended daily allowance. You'll also find folate, vitamin A, iron, potassium, vitamin B6, magnesium, and riboflavin in broccoli. Additionally, broccoli has strong anti-diabetic action, lowering and balancing blood sugars. Broccoli also strengthens the blood and your immune system, improves digestion, lowers cholesterol, and helps in weight loss.

Spinach

Spinach may have been good for Popeye, but it's even better for you. Spinach has high quantities of vitamin A, folate, iron, magnesium, calcium, vitamin C, riboflavin, potassium, and vitamin B6. It's also a great source of fiber, not to mention its anti-diabetic effect. It also improves blood pressure, blood quality, digestion, and immunity— all while lowering cholesterol and helping in weight loss.

Vegetables aren't the only source of these great nutrients. Whatever can be said about vegetables can also be said about grasses. Grasses are incredibly nutrient dense, even more so than vegetables. Just two examples characterize the health benefits of grass:

Wheat grass

More than 100 food elements, including every identified mineral and trace mineral as well as the vitamin B complex, can be found in wheat grass. It is also rich in vitamins C, E, and K, and has one of the highest levels of vitamin A of any food. Not only that, but wheat grass is also 25 percent protein and contains high amounts of an antifungal/antimycotoxin called laetrile.

Barley grass

Barely grass has seven times more vitamin C than oranges and four times as much thiamine (vitamin B) than whole wheat flour and 30 times as much as milk.

Ingredients to look for in green drinks:

Green Kamut Grass • Barley Grass • Lemon Grass • Shave Grass • Wheat Grass • Couch Grass • Oat Grass • Watercress Herb • Sage Leaf • Thyme Leaf • Aloe Vera Leaf Concentrate • Broccoli Floret • Turmeric Rhizome • Tomato Fruit • Billberry Leaf • Alfalfa Leaf Juice • Dandelion Leaf • Black Walnut Leaf • Plantain Leaf • Red Raspberry Leaf • Boldo Leaf • Golden Seal Leaf • Papaya Leaf • Strawberry Leaf • Rosemary Leaf • Blueberry Leaf • Kale Leaf • Peppermint Leaf • Spearmint Leaf • Wintergreen Leaf • Soy Lecithin • Blackberry Leaf • Mineral Mix • White Willow Bark • Slippery Elm Bark • Marshmallow Root • Pau d'arco Bark • Cornsilk • Beta Carotene • Rose Hips Fruit • Echinacea Tops • Meadowsweet Herb • Soy Sprouts • Okra Fruit • Cabbage Herb • Spinach Leaf • Celery Seed • Parsley • Alfalfa Leaf

While ensuring that you eat the proper vegetables and grasses is a good step in the right direction, drinking them in the form of a green drink is even better. A green drink literally takes the benefits of pounds of vegetables and green foods and makes them available in a drinkable blend. In other words, with a green drink you're getting more bang for the buck.

THE 2ND FOUNDATION STONE: ALKALIZED AND ENERGIZED WATER

Your body is 70 percent water. Water composes 70 percent of muscle, 25 percent of fats, 75 percent of your brain, and over 90 percent of your blood. Water regulates your body's temperature, cushions and protects vital organs, aids in digestion, transports nutrients within each cell, and dispels wastes. Water also helps to prevent kidney stones caused by the body combining excess acid with calcium. One study also showed that women who drank more than five glasses of water a day had a 45 percent less risk of colon cancer. Yet another study showed a decreased chance of bladder cancer when more than 2.5 quarts of fluid were consumed daily. Maintaining your level of hydration is very important to the overall health of your pancreas and your body as a whole. You should be drinking at least four liters of water—or about one gallon—per day.

Dehydration Dangers

We're aware that extreme dehydration can result in death. What many of us don't know is that even mild dehydration can have terrible effects on the body's performance:

• A 3 percent drop in body weight through water loss causes a 10 percent drop of contractile strength in your muscles and an 8 percent drop of speed, as well as losses in muscular endurance.

• A 4 percent loss can cause dizziness, and you can experience as much as a 30 percent drop in your capacity for physical labor.

• A 5 percent loss will cause problems with concentration, drowsiness, impatience, and headaches.

• A 6 percent loss will cause your heart to race and your body's temperature regulation mechanism to fail.

• A 7 percent loss will lead to collapse.

Drink Enough Water

In an average day—one that doesn't feature physical activity, extreme environmental conditions, or a few other water-draining factors such as air travel or high-rise buildings—you can experience a 1 percent loss of water. Many of us have at least a few factors that contribute to water loss in our lives. We may not travel in an airplane every day, but if you're health conscious you're working out-a major dehydrating activity. You may also live in a hot or dry (or even worse, both) environment. How much more dehydrated are you because of these factors?

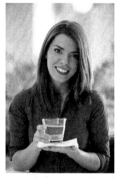

A recent study conducted by the Yankelovich Partners for the Nutrition Information Center at the New York Hospital, Cornell Medical Center, and the International Bottled Water Association revealed that dehydration is a much more wide-spread problem than you may have thought.

"Most Americans are probably only getting about one-third of the valuable hydration benefits they need," explains Barbara Levine, R.D., Ph.D., Director of the Nutrition Information Center at the New York Hospital, Cornell Medical Center. "The vast majority isn't drinking enough water to begin with, and to make matters worse, many don't realize that beverages containing alcohol and caffeine actually rob the body of water."

A study conducted at the Nutrition Information Center reports many other startling facts:

• The average American only consumes 4.6 servings of water a day; barely half of the recommended amount.

• Only one in five meets the recommended eight 8-ounce glasses of water a day.

• 44 percent of respondents reported drinking three or fewer servings of water daily.

• Nearly one in 10 respondents reported drinking no water at all!

"It's troubling that so few Americans drink the recommended amount of water daily," notes Levine. "The consumption of water and other hydrating beverages is crucial for proper retention and use of the body's water in complex and intricate biochemical processes." Not so surprising is the overwhelming ignorance of the effects of dehydration. Survey respondents were aware that mild dehydration could cause dry skin and headaches, but the knowledge seems to stop there.

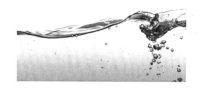

• One in five did not know that caffeinated beverages dehydrate.

• Nearly half—47 percent—of Americans are unaware that they lose as much water when asleep as when awake.

• 37 percent do not know that the body needs as much water in cold weather as it does in warm.

"This look at America's hydration habits suggests what could be a significant and widespread health concern," reports Levine. "The survey clearly demonstrates the need for much more public education about the benefits of proper hydration and the problems even minor dehydration can cause."

Drink the Right Water

Keeping your body properly hydrated is not just a matter of drinking the right amount of water. It's just as important to drink the right water.

Our water supplies today have become increasingly contaminated and thus dangerous to our health. But just as water can be ruined by certain additives and actions, so too can it be made healthier. By drinking alkalized and energized water, you will rehydrate and revitalize your body.

Pure water ranks an even seven on the pH scale. However, often tap water and even some bottled waters are actually acidic. When water is acidic it could contain

metal ions such as iron, lead, cadmium and mercury—all toxic, and, in excess, can cause serious health issues.

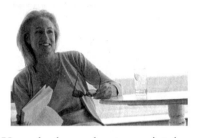

Your body seeks to maintain a slightly alkaline state. When we introduce acidic substances into our body, we throw that alkaline state off. Your body doesn't want that. So, in an effort to overcome that situation, your body will use alkaline substances to counteract the acidic ones.

Now that the acid is neutralized, you'll need to wash it away. How do you do that? With water. Pure water, which is neutral, would wash away those wastes. Unfortunately, our water today has been contaminated and changed to the point where it is more acidic than neutral. What would happen if you try to wash away an acid with an acid? With acidic water, your body has to employ even more alkaline substances to balance out the problems.

Contrast that practice with the idea of drinking alkaline water. By drinking alkaline water, you are helping your body to maintain its preferred alkaline state. You'll also help prevent the gleaning of alkaline substances from other body parts. Alkaline water is also highly oxygenated; oxygen is perhaps the single most important substance that your body needs. Finally, microforms won't be able to thrive in an environment that is supplied with alkaline water. Here's a brief list of some of the benefits of alkaline water:

• Alkaline water ranks at 8.5 to 9.5 on the pH scale. That's 1.5 to 2.5 points of alkalinity that can be used to counteract acids. Take cola, for instance. Cola comes in at 2.5 on the pH scale—4.5 points of acidity. Mix cola and alkaline water together and they begin to cancel each other out,

• Your body can only absorb ionic minerals. That's fortunate as these minerals include calcium, magnesium, and potassium—all of which are required by the body and are alkaline. Alkaline water is filled with these minerals, whereas more acidic beverages have minerals such as copper, iron, manganese, phosphorous, cadmium, and lead.

• Water molecules form clusters. Tap water has about 10-20 molecules per cluster. Alkaline water, however, has 5-6 molecules per cluster, making it "wetter" with lower surface tension. This enables alkaline water to better penetrate body tissues.

Alkaline water is indeed powerful when it comes to affecting the health of your body. Not only is it a more effective hydrator, but it also counteracts the effects of acidity. Counteracting these effects also means preventing degenerative diseases linked to over-acidification of your body, such as:

- Heart disease
- Osteoporosis
- Gallstones
- High blood pressure
- Kidney stones
- Tooth decay

Even more pertinent to our subject, alkaline water can help prevent obesity and diabetes. In a recent investigation in Norway, a possible link was found between acidic drinking water and type I diabetes. Children who consumed water with a pH between 6.2 and 6.9 were nearly four times more likely to be diagnosed with type I diabetes compared to children drinking less acidic water.

Alkalizing water is only half of the battle. You also need to energize it. Electro-magnetic microionization is quite a mouthful to say. It's also a process of energizing water. The process of energizing water through this electro-magnetic microionization involves increasing the amount of electrons in water. This, in turn, neutralizes excess gastrointestinal, respiratory, and metabolic acids associated with hypoglycemia and diabetes. The most critical need for a diabetic is to correct the loss of electrons in blood, urine, and saliva. The vital importance of adding these electrons to your system is impossible to ignore.

If your blood is found to be oxidized—lacking electrons—by more than two units on the rH2 scale (a measurement of oxidation that ranges from 0 to 44, with 22 being a healthy, non-diabetic person), you have 100 times fewer electrons than a healthy individual. This results in low energy levels.

If you come in at over 25, you're probably suffering from hypoglycemia or chronic fatigue and diabetes. These high levels of oxidation are often associated with high levels of tissue acidity, indicating a generalized increase in tissue aging-literally making you feel older than you actually are! But you can reclaim your health by simply ensuring you are drinking enough alkalized and energized water. When people begin drinking the right kind of water, biological age and oxidative stress fall, and their acid/alkaline balance levels out to where it should be.

THE 3RD FOUNDATION STONE: PH DROPS

Alkalized and energized water can do wonders for your health, but if you want to work miracles, you'll need to add in pH drops.

pH drops are basically a sodium chlorite additive that you can put into your water. The pH drops act as oxygen and electron catalyst,

bringing more oxygen and electrons into your blood and thus to your body's cells. The sodium chlorite in the pH drops has been shown to alkalize, energize, oxygenate, and balance a diabetic's acidic blood, tissues, and organs, including the pancreas.

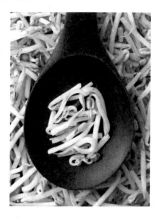

THE 4TH FOUNDATION STONE SOY SPROUTS

Sprouts are just about the best food you can eat. Filled with vitamins, minerals, and complete proteins, they are also high in enzymes, nucleic acids, and vitamin B12. Isoflavones in soy sprouts have been shown to lower cholesterol and inhibit atherosclerosis-a leading cause of cardiovascular disease and a great support to the pancreas in its exocrine and endocrine activities.

The vitamin B12 that naturally occurs in sprouts has also been the inspiration of many recent studies. A preliminary trial, conducted in 1995 and reported in the review journal Current Therapeutic Research, found people with nerve damage due to kidney dysfunction or to diabetes plus kidney disease experienced a significant reduction of nerve pain and a significant improvement of nerve function when their diets were supplemented with vitamin B12. The incredible benefits of soy, including lowering blood cholesterol levels, balancing sugar levels, inhibiting atherosclerosis, preventing cancer and osteoporosis, and the amelioration of menopausal symptoms, can all be found in soy sprouts as well.

THE 5TH FOUNDATION STONE MARINE LIPIDS AND BORAGE OIL

With the increased awareness of health also came a conspicuous error. We've been taught to lump all fats into the "bad" category. Such is not the case. Your body actually needs some fats to live and function properly they are, as their name states, essential. In fact, some fats can actually help improve your health.

If you want to avoid the unhealthy fats, eliminate the long-chained saturated and partially hydrogenated fats so prolific in the American diet. The healthy unsaturated fats should be a part of your diet. Polyunsaturated fats should make up 20 to 40 percent of your caloric intake. Flax, borage, evening primrose, grape seed, and hemp oils are good sources of these fats. Most oils contain both monounsaturated and polyunsaturated fats. Olive oil, raw nuts, and avocados are beneficial sources of monounsaturated fats. But make sure the oils are cold pressed (extracted and packaged without using heat.) Heating the oil breaks it down, robbing it of its benefits.

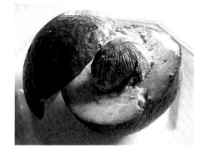

Essential fats have many uses in your body. They strengthen white blood cells, lubricate joints, insulate the body against heat loss, provide energy, and are used to make hormone-like prostaglandins that protect against heart disease, stroke, high blood pressure, atherosclerosis, blood clots, and diabetes. They can help relieve secondary symptoms of diabetes such as arthritis, asthma, PMS, allergies, skin conditions, diabetic neuropathy, kidney dysfunction, hypercholesterolemia, and some behavior disorders. They also improve brain function.

But the benefits don't stop there. Essential fats are used in a number of different processes in your body, including cellular regeneration and growth. EPA and DHA are two of the most used forms of essential fats. They are abundant in brain cells, nerve relay stations, visual receptors, adrenal glands, and sex glands. They have also been shown to prevent diabetes, osteoporosis, cancer, cardiovascular disease, and stroke.

The best sources of the essential fats that your body needs are marine lipids and borage oil. Marine lipids are an excellent source of the omega 3 fatty acids EPA and DHA. Borage oil provides a natural source of gamma linolenic acid, linolenic acid, and erucic acid, which protect your body's insulin-producing beta cells from acid breakdown. They also provide the needed fats for building the bi-lipid membrane of every cell in your body.

CHAPTER 6
HOW FOUNDATION STONES AFFECT DIABETES

Sure, these foundation stones are great for overall health, but what do they have to do with diabetes? Everything. Diabetes is a reflection of your body's inability to process sugars or effectively use insulin. This problem stems from damage—largely the damage caused by over-acidification. The pancreas is one of the many body parts that are susceptible to acid damage. And with no redundancy program in place—meaning your body doesn't have a back-up plan when insulin fails—you'll be in a great deal of trouble when the pancreas stops working.

Not only that, but cells can grow resistant to insulin. This happens because of one simple fact: a diabetic's cells are exposed to too much insulin too often. The cause? Our poor diets. Our bloodstreams are overloaded with sugar, and to counteract that our bodies increase insulin production. To fix this problem, we need to lower our blood sugar levels and provide our bodies with fuel that is both healthy and economical.

These foundation stones address both problems. With the added nutrients of these supplements, our bodies will be able to repair and rebuild. But that's not all. You'll notice that your energy levels will increase while taking these supplements. You'll feel more enthused, energetic, excited—more alive! That's because you are. The foundation stones can breathe new life into your body.

BURN FAT, NOT SUGAR

When you over-exercise or exercise anaerobically, you put your body's approximate 75 trillion cells at risk not for gain, but for loss. Look at some of the athletes we assumed to be healthy and fit like Jim Fix, the marathon runner, or Florence "Flo Jo" Joyner; both died from heart attacks. You hear about athletes every year who die on and off the track, field, or court.

On the other hand there is Stu Mittleman, an Ultra Marathon runner and world record holder. Stu ran across America doing the equivalent of two marathons a day, every day for 57 days. He did this without the side effects of excess acid. How? Stu understood the importance of burning fat rather than sugar. He also drank his greens and good fats while running. The idea of carbohydrate-loading before a physical event is physiological suicide. The optimal game plan is to burn fat rather than sugar. Burning fat produces twice the energy or electrons with half the acid versus burning or breaking down sugar or protein to release their electrons. This is significant when you are trying to increase electron energy and move acids out of the body at the same time. The key to healthful exercise, especially for diabetics, is to never go to pain. If you're in pain, you're burning sugar, which places you squarely in a state of acidosis. If you reach this point, you should stop immediately and start alkalizing by drinking your green drink and alkalized/energized water.

Here are a few physical and emotional signs that will tell you when you're burning sugar instead of fat:

- *Feeling light-headed*
- *Burning sensations in your body*
- *Dizziness*
- *Cannot carry on a conversation while exercising*
- *Cloudy thinking*
- *Cold hands or feet*
- *Your brow is furrowed and tight*
- *Tingling in the extremities*
- *Your fists are clenched tightly*

- *Peripheral vision narrows*
- *Your muscles are tight*
- *You can hear yourself breathing*
- *You have a knot in your throat*
- *Inhaling and exhaling through your mouth instead of your nose*
- *You become agitated or anxious*
- *Your sweat smells like ammonia*
- *You become disconnected with your environment*
- *You feel systemic or localized pain in your body*

In comparison, when you're burning fat rather than sugar you will experience the following physical and emotional signs:

- *You have a peaceful feeling*
- *Your facial expressions are relaxed and happy*
- *You feel grounded*

- *Your peripheral vision is widened*
- *You feel connected to your external environment*
- *All your senses are enhanced*
- *You are inhaling and exhaling through your nose not your mouth*
- *You feel no pain*
- *You have a sense of euphoria*
- *Your breathing is quiet and easy*
- *Your mind is clear*
- *You feel more flexible*
- *You can carry on a conversation while exercising*
- *You feel "in the zone"*

Choosing to burn fat as your main source of fuel for energy in life and especially during exercise will minimize acidity, increase energy and vitality, increase strength and endurance, improve the performance of all bodily functions, and extend the quality and quantity of your life.

Exercising aerobically without pain will help you remove acids from your body fluids and tissues and will help provide the alkaline environment necessary for regeneration and healthy body function.

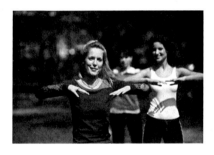

CHAPTER 7
REDUCE STRESS IN
YOUR BODY

All of us live with a certain amount of stress each day. Our relationships and jobs cause us stress. Driving down the road and narrowly missing an accident cause stress. Confrontations, concerns, and illness can all produce stress. Common forms of stress are anxiety; overwork; inadequate diet, sleep, or exercise; trauma; injury; emotional pressures; and exposure to outside contaminates. Regardless of what causes it or how big a stressor is, our bodies react in the same way. It's a holdover from evolution, and we call it the fight or flight response.

When your body reacts to stress, it does so by releasing certain hormones designed to equip your body with the tools it needs to fight or flee. These hormones prepare your body for emergency action, starring with the cardiovascular system. They constrict the arteries, making your heart beat faster in order to rush more blood to your muscles and brain. Blood is also drawn back from the skin, and the clotting time is quickened so that your body will bleed less if injured. Under stress, your body also raises the white blood-cell count to help keep the internal environment clean.

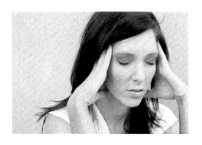

The reaction then moves into your metabolism. Red blood-cell counts are increased to deliver more oxygen to your body's cells so that they can burn fuel faster. The supply of fuel is also increased by stimulating the liver and muscles to release sugar into the bloodstream. When blood-sugar levels increase, your pancreas reacts by pouring more insulin into the blood, enabling the excess sugar to enter cells.

Now consider this. The fight or flight response was not meant to be left on continuously. Imagine your vehicle. When you want that little burst of speed needed to pass another car or make it up a hill, your car will mount up to the challenge with only minimal damage. Now imagine keeping your gas pedal floored all the time without ever shutting off your car. Complicate things even more by leaving the parking brake on. What will happen to your car? Eventually something will break down.

The world we live in leaves us in a state of constant stress. In effect, our gas pedals are constantly floored. Unfortunately, we hold back the fight or flight response, giving our bodies no place to vent that built-up power. In other words, we leave our parking brake on. Something is going to give. That something involves your pancreas and the insulin response. Constant, continued stress is a vicious cycle that can lead to a host of diabetic symptomatologies, including hyperglycemia, hyperinsulemia, obesity, underweight, insulin resistivity, diabetes, and even pancreatic cancer.

Fortunately, this is an easily rectifiable situation. Regular aerobic exercise is critical for diabetics and pre-diabetics. Adequate exercise lowers blood pressure and serum triglycerides as well as insulin levels. Exercise is also vital in controlling blood sugar levels. Most of these benefits are accomplished with exercise as easy as a regular brisk walk.

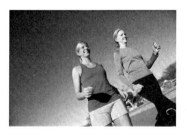

CHAPTER 8
MAINTAINING THE PH BALANCE

Proper nutrition and weight maintenance are only the beginning of the battle against diabetes. Your body strives to maintain a number of balances. Temperature, for instance, is a vital balance that your body works to maintain. Slight variations above or below the normal 98.6 degrees Fahrenheit can result in serious problems-even death. But even as important as this balance is, there is a more critical balance for your body-the pH balance.

The pH scale is a measure of acidity and alkalinity. On a scale of 1 to 14, with 7 being neutral, pH represents how acidic or alkaline a substance is. When acids and alkalines meet in certain ratios, they cancel each other out. Your body seeks to maintain a pH level of 7.365, which is slightly alkaline. With the exception of certain body systems—specifically the stomach and colon—your body will try to maintain that alkaline pH level.

The importance of maintaining the pH balance becomes clear when you understand the effects of acidification on your pancreas. When your body registers that it is becoming acidic, it will take measures to counteract the problem. Normally, your body has stores of alkaline substances, such as sodium, potassium, calcium, and magnesium, that it can employ to help regain an alkaline state. However, when sufficient amounts of these substances are not present, either because of malnutrition or over-acidification, your body will start to pull alkaline minerals from other areas, such as calcium from your bones or magnesium from your muscles. Unfortunately, these areas need those minerals as well and are weakened by the gleaning that your body is forced to do in order to maintain its pH balance.

One of those areas that suffer from this acidification process is the pancreas. In early stages of imbalance, symptoms may not be very serious.

However, as the imbalance continues, the complications become more serious. Your pancreas and other organs become weakened and body systems will start to fail. Eventually, the over-acidification causes oxygen levels in your body to drop, which in turn stops metabolism. In other words, cells begin to die, which means you begin to die as well.

When your pancreas begins to fail, insulin production also plummets. Thus diabetes enters the scene. But if you can reverse the damage caused by over-acidification, your pancreas can bounce back.

Diabetes isn't the only problem caused by this over-acidification. Many microforms thrive in the created acidic environment, and their presence is detrimental to your health.

To correct this problem, you need to help your body return to its slightly alkaline state of 7.365. As your body begins to return to this desired state, those troublesome microforms will be brought under control, and many of the symptoms you may be suffering from-which are actually warning signals from your body that something is wrong-will disappear. It's very similar to stagnant water. When you return water to a flowing state, mosquitoes cannot reproduce and are forced to go elsewhere. Bacteria, yeast, fungus, and mold can't live in an alkaline environment, so they are forced to return to their normal, balanced state.

You can help your body regain its homeostasis-or balanced state-by providing it with the alkaline substances that it needs and by avoiding those substances that promote an acidic state. The nutrition and supplementation plans that we've already discussed will go a long way toward overcoming this problem. The ultimate key to all of this, however, is you. You have to make the decision that you will change your health-and your life-for the better. No plan works without you doing your part.

CHAPTER 9
POWER OF SUPPLEMENTS

Did you know that supplements can help prevent, treat, and even cure diabetes and obesity?

Diabetes is not the natural state of your body. Nature intended for your body to be healthy, perhaps that's why she provided a few supplemental plants and nutrients to help battle the disease.

MIRACLE MINERALS
Montmorillonite

Geophagy, according to Taber's Cyclopedia Medical Dictionary, is "a condition in which the patient eats inedible substances, such as chalk or earth." Another term, pica, is defined as "a perversion of appetite with craving for substances not fit for food, such as clay, ashes, or plaster." This craving, once you understand what Montmorillonite can do for you, is not a "perversion of appetite." Rather, it's a logical course to take if you want incredible health. This may surprise you, but clay can provide your body with an impressive assortment of minerals, including calcium, iron, magnesium, potassium, manganese, sodium, and silica-all alkalizing and foundational to the production of other elements of your body.

The minerals in clay exist in natural proportion to one another. This encourages their absorption by the intestinal villi. Oxygen, silica, and potassium exist as spheres arranged in a regular three-dimensional pattern in edible clay. The spheres are the building blocks of the clay minerals, and the arrangement of the spheres determines the type of mineral.

Edible clay has been credited with improving the health of many people suffering from a wide range of illnesses, including:

Constipation • Diarrhea • Anemia • Chronic infections • Skin ailments (such as eczema and acne) • Heavy metal poisoning • Exposure to pesticides and other acidic toxins • Arthritis • Acid reflux • Infertility• Liver disease • Obesity • Hair loss • Type I and type II diabetes

Among the clays suitable for eating, Montmorillonite is the most common and the most sought after. The particles of Montmorillonite clay carry a negative electrical charge, whereas impurities or toxins carry a positive charge. For this very reason, Montmorillonite clay has been used to absorb the colloidal impurities in beer, wine, liquor, and cider. The impurities in these liquids can be chelated or coagulated and then removed by stirring in small amounts of Montmorillonite clay.

This process also works in the body. When Montmorillonite is taken internally, the positively charged exotoxins and mycotoxins are attracted to the negatively charged Montmorillonite particles. An exchange reaction occurs, and the acidic toxin is held in suspension until the body can eliminate both particles.

Geoghagy Benefits

Here are a few things people reported after eating Montmorillonite clay for two to four weeks:

Well-regulated bowel • Relief from constipation • Better, sounder sleep • No more indigestion • No more depression • weight loss • Reduction in insulin use • No more ulcers •No more acne • No more dandruff • Hair growing back • Better digestion • Increase in energy • Less "wandering pain" all over the body • clearer skin • Whiter, brighter eyes • More alert and clear-headed • Emotional uplift • Tension relief • Enhanced growth and tissue repair of gums and skin • More effective immune system

Montmorillonite clay works on the entire organisms—inside and out. No one part of the body is left untouched by its healing energies.

NADHP

NADHP is an acronym that stands for B-nicotinamide adenine dinucleotide phosphate-the H is for a highly active hydrogen ion. This reduced form of Coenzyme 1 reacts with oxygen to produce, in a cascade of reactions, water and energy. This electron energy is stored in the form of adenosine triphosphate, or ATP. In other words, NADHP-derived from splitting our food-combines with molecular oxygen present in all living cells to form water and energy. One molecule of NADHP yields three molecules of ATP. The more NADHP a cell has available, the more energy it can produce. Without NADHP, energy cannot be produced, and lactic acid is formed. Lactic acid is one of the primary acids that lead to diabetes, obesity, and cancer and its many related symptomatologies.

This compound is present in all our cells, but it is vitally important to the energy production of the brain, heart, and nerves. Heart cells contain approximately 90 micrograms of NADHP per gram of tissue. Brain cells contain approximately 50 micrograms per gram of tissue.

Chromium

Chromium is an essential mineral that stimulates the activity of enzymes involved in the metabolism of glucose for energy and the synthesis of fatty acids and cholesterol. Chromium appears to increase the effectiveness of insulin and its ability to handle glucose, thus preventing hypoglycemia or diabetes. In the blood, it competes with iron in the transport of protein. Chromium may also be involved in the synthesis of protein, through its binding action with RNA molecules.

In 1957, two researchers, Swartz and Mertz, recognized that chromium is a very important factor in maintaining proper glucose metabolism.

When they gave this substance to laboratory rats with glucose intolerance—a prediabetic condition marked by impaired ability to metabolize carbohydrates—significant improvements in sugar metabolism resulted.

A 1993 study involving 243 diabetics taking 200 micrograms a day of chromium revealed similar results. These patients were aware of the fact that they were taking chromium and were told to reduce their oral hypoglycemic medication, insulin, as needed in order to avoid hypoglycemic episodes. More than half of the people with type II diabetes and more than one-third of those with type I were able to cut back on their medications.

A much larger study was conducted by the US Department of Agriculture's Human Nutrition Research Center at the Beijing Medical University, China in 1997. Researchers divided 180 type II diabetics into three groups. Each group was assigned to take 100 micrograms of chromium picolinate, 500 micrograms of chromium picolinate, or a placebo respectively twice a day. No other changes were made in their medications, diets, or activity levels. When their blood-sugar levels were tested after four months, the patients taking chromium had reductions in blood sugar, insulin, cholesterol, and glycosylated hemoglobin. Those taking 500 micrograms had even greater reductions than those on lower levels.

Two of the most compelling studies on chromium and weight loss were conducted by Dr. Gilbert R. Kaats. In his most recent study, published in June 1998, 122 subjects were given 400 micrograms of chromium picolinate per day or a placebo. After 90 days, adjusting for caloric intake and expenditure, Kaats determined that the chromium did indeed have positive effects on weight and body composition. Those taking chromium lost more weight (an average of 17.1 pounds compared to 3.9 pounds for the placebo group), fat mass (16.9 pounds versus 3.3 pounds), and percentage of body fat (6.3 percent versus 1.2 percent).

Adding supplemental chromium to your diet has benefits. Ensuring that your body has a sufficient amount of chromium, however, is vital. Even a slight chromium deficiency will have serious effects on your body. Tests indicate systematic deficiency of chromium is common in the United States a rare occurrence in other countries. Americans tend to be deficient because our soil does not contain an adequate supply, and thus chromium cannot be absorbed by the crops or reach the water supply. The refining of foods is another probable cause of chromium loss. Government surveys suggest that most Americans fail to get even 50 micrograms of chromium a day.

A chromium deficiency may be a factor that can upset the function of insulin and result in depressed growth rates and severe glucose intolerance in diabetics. Researchers also believe that the interaction of chromium and insulin is not limited to glucose metabolism, but also applies to amino acid metabolism. Chromium may inhibit the formation of aortic plaques, and a deficiency may very well contribute to arteriosclerosis.

Vanadium

Vanadium is a trace mineral that research has established as an effective supplement in reversing diabetes. Numerous animal studies and a growing body of human research show that vanadium improves fasting glucose levels and is effective in controlling blood sugar.

In a 1996 study, eight men and women with type II diabetes received 50 milligrams of vanadyl sulfate—a form of vanadium —twice a day for four weeks. This was followed by a placebo for four weeks. A 20-percent average reduction in fasting glucose levels was recorded. Interestingly, this reduction extended into the placebo period.

Recent research suggests that vanadium acts in a manner very similar to insulin. Vanadium is one of the few compounds, other than insulin, that can activate GLUT-4 transporters—the substances that carry glucose from the surface of the cell to the cell's interior. In essence, vanadium mimics the action of insulin.

Magnesium

An essential mineral, magnesium accounts for about .05 percent of the body's total weight. Nearly 70 percent of the body's supply of magnesium is located in the bones. The final 30 percent is found in the soft tissues and body fluids.

Magnesium is involved in many essential metabolic processes. It activates enzymes necessary for the metabolism of carbohydrates and amino acids; plays an important role in neuromuscular contractions; helps regulate the acid alkaline balance; promotes absorption and metabolism of other minerals such as calcium, phosphorus, sodium, and potassium; and it helps utilize the B-complex vitamins and vitamin E in the body. Magnesium also helps with bone growth and is necessary for proper functioning of the nerves in muscles, including the heart.

Among many other therapies, magnesium has been effective in treating diabetes, pancreatitis, nervousness, diarrhea, and vomiting. Medical literature contains many studies showing that diabetic patients have below average blood levels of magnesium and higher urinary losses of this mineral. Direct evidence suggesting how important magnesium is in protecting us from cardiovascular disease is offered by reputable scientific studies. Examination of autopsy specimens from cattle that died from magnesium deficiencies clearly indicates obvious cardiovascular degeneration. Heggtveit discovered a decreased magnesium content in the left ventricle of infracted hearts compared to controlled hearts in sudden traumatic deaths. Laurendeau has also seen lower levels of magnesium in the hearts of patients with myocardial necrosis-an occurrence much more noticeable in diabetics. A landmark study by Dr. P. McNair revealed that diabetics with the lowest magnesium levels have the most severe retinopathy. Dr. McNair further concluded that low magnesium levels were more significantly linked to retinopathy than any other factor. It only stands to reason that the diabetic patients put on magnesium supplementation will see an increase in blood and cellular levels of magnesium, thus lowering the risk factor of cardiovascular complications and blindness.

Zinc

Zinc is fast becoming recognized as an essential nutrient. Among its many other good qualities, zinc is an important part of the structure of insulin and influences the secretion of several other body hormones. Deficiencies may cause poor memory, dark skin pigmentation, slow wound healing, sexual difficulties, aching joints, hair loss, and many pancreatic disorders.

Zinc performs a variety of functions in the human body. It is associated with the normal absorption and action of most vitamins, especially the B-complex. It is a constituent of at least 25 enzymes involved in digestion and metabolism. Zinc is a part of the enzyme vital to the formation of insulin. It is also necessary for carbohydrate digestion and phosphorous metabolism. Additionally, it is crucial for the creation of nucleic acids, which control the formation of cellular protein. Zinc is essential for normal growth and proper development of the reproductive organs and for correct functioning of the prostate gland.

From limiting cholesterol deposits to helping in the rapid healing of wounds, zinc has many other uses in the body. Most pertinent to this discussion, however, is zinc's benefit to the diabetic. Zinc has a regulatory effect on insulin in the blood. Adding zinc to insulin prolongs its effect on blood sugar.

A diabetic pancreas contains only about half as much zinc as a healthy, nondiabetic pancreas. Zinc supplementation for diabetics certainly makes sense.

HERBS HELP HEAL

There are certain herbal supplements that, when blended together, can provide the best aid Mother Nature can supply.

As a supplement, this blend provides sound functional support to the physiological systems involved, and in many cases may lessen the need for insulin. It may even ameliorate pre-diabetic or diabetic conditions in many individuals. Beyond that effect, however, the blend invigorates several of the body's most important organs, glands, and glandular organs, especially the liver, pancreas, kidneys, and gallbladder. Used regularly-together with green drinks, green foods, and alkalized and energized water-the effect of these herbs can be extraordinary.

The following herbs are considered to be the primary herbs or active ingredients that make this supplemental blend so effective in the prevention, reversal, and cure of type I and type II diabetes.

Uva Ursi

Uva ursi contains a group of compounds called phenolic glycosides that have been used since the 13th century for their diuretic and urinary anti-septic actions. This activity helps relieve pain from bladder stones; and relieves cystitis, nepritis, and kidney stones. Early in American history, uva ursi was thought to be of great benefit in numerous ailments, as an astringent and anti-scorbutic, and was used as a food. Today, the herb is used as a tonic, specifically in cases involving weakened liver, kidneys, pancreas, and other glands.

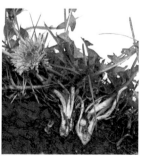

Dandelion Root

Dandelion root exhibits hypoglycemic effects in experimental animals. Some researchers believe that the insulin content of dandelion contains insulin-like principles that may actually substitute for insulin, on a limited basis. More tests need to be done, but it is an interesting hypothesis. The more probable explanation is that because inulin is a concentrated source of dietary fiber, it buffers blood glucose levels, preventing sudden and severe fluctuations. In addition, it benefits diabetics by improving kidney function, especially the kidney's ability to cleanse the blood and reabsorb nutrients. Dandelion's beneficial effects on liver complaints are also important. Research has shown that dandelion stimulates bile production and helps the body get rid of excess water produced by an overly acidic liver. Dandelion extracts have also been reported to benefit the spleen and improve the health of the pancreas.

Parsley

Parsley is commonly used to treat jaundice and gallstones. Though many properties of parsley have been experimentally established (laxative, hypotensive, antacid, and uterine properties), its effects on the liver have not been thoroughly investigated. However, the claims of clinical physicians over the past 100 years reveal parsley to be very effective in remedying an overly acidic liver.

Gentian Root

Gentian root has a focused activity on the glands and organs involved in digestion, such as the gallbladder and the pancreas, with secondary effects on other organs such as the liver and kidneys. Experiments have found that gentian root promotes the secretion of bile. Other experiments recorded gentian root's anti-inflammatory and antacid properties. Diabetics and pre-diabetics will experience increased pancreatic support when taking gentian root. Gentian root may also delay the onset of brittle diabetes-or prevent its occurrence altogether. It also works to delay or prevent heartburn, gastritis, various forms of upset stomach, and even cancer. Gentian root is regarded as one of the premier herbs to use today.

Huckleberry Leaf

Huckleberry leaf is used by many naturopathic physicians to

treat sugar diabetes and ailments of the kidneys and gallbladder. This is not surprising since huckleberry is a close cousin to uva ursi. Its leaves contain very similar compounds. The active principle is neomyrtilcine. The herb is one of the best for mild diabetics and may be especially beneficial for use in "senile" diabetes.

Raspberry Leaf

Raspberry leaves are primarily used for diarrhea and for problems associated with the female biology, but they are also frequently used in folk medicine to relieve urethral and kidney irritation. There is some experimental evidence that raspberry leaf can be used to treat diabetes because of its proven hypoglycemic action.

Bruchu Leaf

Bruchu leaf is aromatic and carminative. It helps to relieve irritation of the bladder, urethra, and kidneys.

Saw Palmetto Berry

Saw palmetto berry, although specific for certain disorders of the prostate and reproductive organs, is generally used effectively for nutritional support of all bodily systems. It helps build new tissue and restore function. Its inclusion in this blend is precisely for the reason that diabetes and other diseases of the glands and organs require the kind of nutritive and biochemical support that these berries provide.

Kelp

Kelp, due to its high iodine content, is a necessary inclusion in any product that purports to help the glands. Kelp contains a sugar named mannitol that imparts some degree of sweetness but does not raise blood sugar levels.

Bladder Rack

Bladder rack, another product of the sea, has been effective against nephritis, bladder inflammation, cardiac degeneration, obesity, thyroid problems, and menstrual problems.

Gymnema Sylvestre

Gymnema sylvestre is a climbing plant native to India. The leaves of this plant have been used in India to treat diabetes for over 2000 years. Chewing the plant also destroys the ability to taste "sweet," resulting in its common Indian name: gur-mar, which means sugar destroyer.

The leaves of this plant work on several fronts to improve diabetic conditions. Some studies suggest that gymnema slows absorption of sugars in the gastrointestinal tract, while others point to its revitalizing effects on the pancreas.

In two studies, researchers gave gymnema sylvestre extract for one or two months to diabetic rats. The number of insulin-secreting beta cells in the rates doubled, and their insulin levels increased to almost normal. This suggests that gymnema stimulates regeneration of important insulin-secreting beta cells in the pancreas. Studies on diabetic rabbits also suggest that gymnema helps sugar get into cells.

Human studies have demonstrated that gymnema has therapeutic value for both typed I and type II diabetes. In one study, individuals with type I diabetes taking an extract for six to eight months had reductions in fasting insulin dose by an average of 23 percent. Furthermore, they were able to cut their insulin dose by an average of 25 percent. In a study of type II diabetes, patients taking 400 mg per day of similar herbal extract for 18 to 20 months also had notable reductions in blood glucose. The most impressive aspect of the study was the 21 of the 22 patients involved were able to significantly reduce their dosages of blood-sugar lowering drugs-five managed to discontinue drug use altogether.

CHAPTER 10
IT'S UP TO YOU

Few things in life are more important that your health. How good or bad your health is will determine, for the most part, what kind of activities you can participate in and how active you can be. Poor health can limit your lifestyle drastically. Illness, diseases, infections, inflammation, depression, lethargy, and lack of desire can all result from poor health.

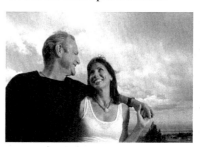

But good nutrition can help to counteract all of that. Providing your body with the needed vitamins and minerals can ensure that you will love a long, productive life, free of diabetes. Good eating habits are so very essential not only to staying alive, but also to living abundantly.

But eating the best possible diet in the world is not an insurance against nutrient deficiencies. Your diet may not be as good as you think. The quality of foods has dropped considerably in the last few decades. Soils are depleted and lacking in vitamins, minerals, and other nutrients. Foods are processed to the point of being robbed of any redeeming virtue. Heated foods lose their nutrients at alarming rates. Popular sources of foods just don't hit the mark when it comes to healthy eating.

That's why supplementation is so very important, especially for the diabetic. The only way to make sure that you are getting all the vitamins, minerals, micronutrients and macronutrients that you need is by enhancing your diet with effective nutritional supplements.

Green drinks provide your body with over 125 vitamins and minerals-the very vitamins and minerals that your body, and specifically your pancreas, needs to protect and heal itself. You'll also find other macronutrients in green powders, like protein and fiber. Beyond that, beneficial herbs, vitamins, minerals, and cell salts can be added to help promote and improve vital pancreatic functions. These herbs cleanse and detoxify the pancreas, strengthen and stimulate the circulatory system, improve digestion, and provide a host of other benefits.

The alternative, of course, is less than desirable. Not only does diabetes place you at twice the risk of death, it also increases your risks of many other complications:

• Heart disease and stroke: Adults with diabetes have heart disease death rates about 2 to 4 times higher than adults without diabetes. The risk for stroke is also 2 to 4 times higher for diabetics. This increased risk accounts for 65 percent of deaths among diabetics.

• High blood pressure: About 73 percent of adults with diabetes have blood pressure equal to or greater than 130/180, or use prescription medications for hypertension.

• Blindness: Diabetes is the leading cause of new cases of blindness among adults 20-74 years old. Diabetic retinopathy causes from 12,000 to 24,000 new cases of blindness each year.

• Kidney disease: Diabetes accounts for 43 percent of new cases of endstage renal disease. In 2000, more than 41,000 people with diabetes began treatment for end-stage renal disease. That same year, 129,183 diabetics underwent dialysis or kidney transplantation.

• Nervous system disease: Between 60 and 70 percent of diabetics have mild to severe forms of nervous system damage. This damage includes impaired sensation or pain in the feet or hands, slowed digestion, carpel tunnel syndrome, and other nerve problems. Severe forms of diabetic nerve disease are a major contributing cause of lower-extremity amputations.

• Amputations: More than 60 percent of nontraumatic lower-limb amputations in the United States occur among people with diabetes.

From 2000 to 2001, about 82,000 nontraumatic lower-limb amputations were performed among people with diabetes.

• Dental disease: Periodontal or gum diseases are more common among people with diabetes than among people without diabetes. Among young adults, those with diabetes are often at twice the risk of those who don't have diabetes. Almost one-third of diabetics have severe periodontal diseases.

• Pregnancy complications: Poorly controlled diabetes before conception and during the first trimester of pregnancy can cause major birth defects in 5 to 10 percent of pregnancies and spontaneous abortions in 15 to 20 percent of pregnancies. During the second and third trimesters, poor control of diabetes can result in excessively large babies, posing a risk to both the mother and the child.

• Other complications: Uncontrolled diabetes often leads to biochemical imbalances that can cause acute life-threatening events such as diabetic ketoacidosis and hyperosmolar (nonketotic) coma. People with diabetes are more susceptible to many other illnesses. Once they acquire these illnesses, they often have worse prognoses than people without diabetes. For example, they are more likely to die with pneumonia or influenza than people who do not have diabetes.

(Statistics taken from the American Diabetes Association National Diabetes Fact Sheet)

The plain truth is that diabetes is just too scary to not do something about this destructive disease. What's truly sad is that many people do not know that there is something they can do.

Now that you know, decide today that you will fight this dreadful disease. Change your life-even if you only do so one tiny step at a time. Work towards being healthier. Implement a nutritious and healthy diet plan. Start being more active. Watch your acid/alkaline balance. Supplement your diet with the foundational stone supplements. You can do it.

Let's work to together to eradicate this terrible disease before it becomes a widespread epidemic.